I0781800

ORAL CANCER DIET COOKBOOK

Nourishing Recipes For Healing, Recovery, And Prevention With Cancer-Fighting Foods, Easy Meal Plans, And Nutritional Guidance

STEPHANIE LOUDER

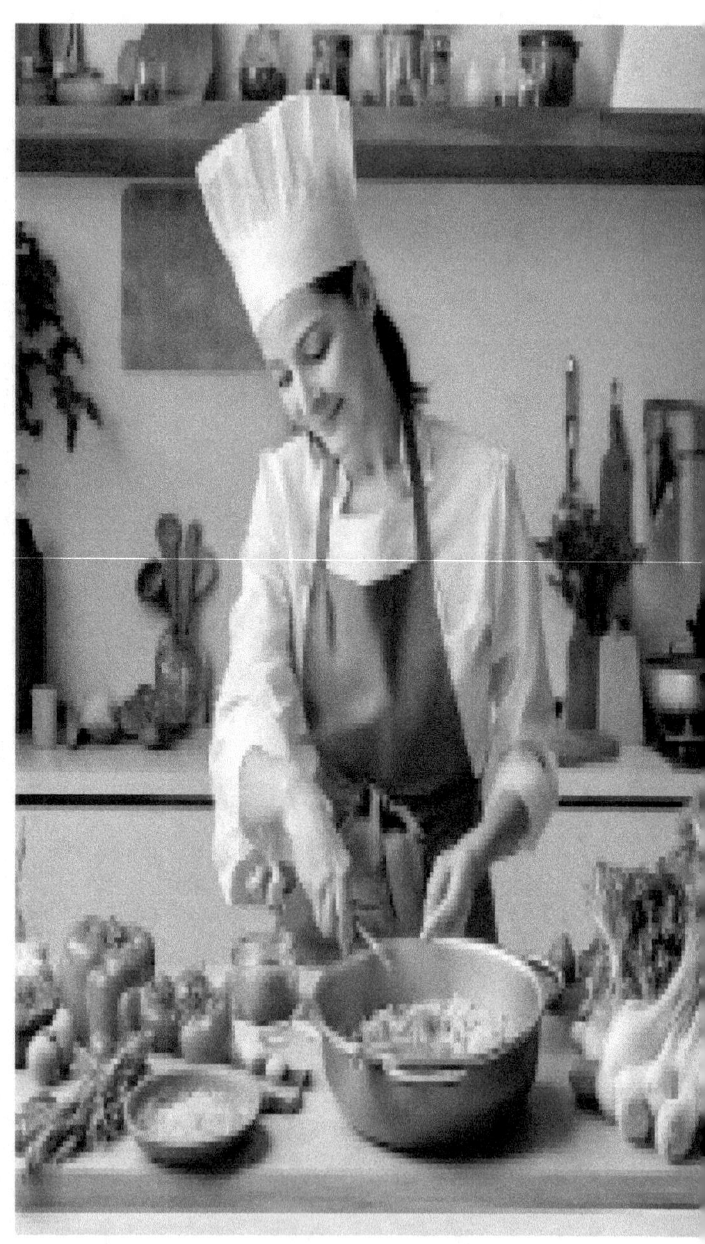

Contents

Copyright © 2024 Stephanie Louder.

All rights reserved.

Unauthorized reproduction or distribution of this material is prohibited. For permissions, contact Stephanie Louder at stephanielouder13@gmail.com

Disclaimer

This book authored by Stephanie Louder, is provided for informational purposes only.

Neither the author nor the publisher assumes any responsibility for the use or misuse of the information herein. This guide does not endorse or support any specific platform or method. Readers are encouraged to consult with healthcare professionals for personalized advice.

CHAPTER 1
Understanding Oral Cancer And Nutrition

Oral cancer is a significant health concern characterized by abnormal cell growth in the mouth, lips, tongue, or throat. It can manifest in various forms, including squamous cell carcinoma, which accounts for the majority of cases.

This type of cancer can affect vital functions such as eating, speaking, and swallowing, making it crucial to address not only with medical treatments but also with a well-rounded approach that includes nutrition. The role of nutrition in oral cancer recovery cannot be overstated, as it plays a pivotal role in supporting overall health, enhancing treatment outcomes, and improving quality of life for patients.

When considering nutrition for oral cancer patients, several key aspects come into play. First and foremost is the need to maintain adequate nutrition despite potential challenges such as difficulty chewing, swallowing problems, or changes in taste and appetite due to treatments like chemotherapy and radiation therapy. A balanced diet that provides essential nutrients is essential for supporting the immune system, promoting tissue healing, and minimizing treatment-related side effects.

Key nutrients play a crucial role in supporting oral cancer patients during their recovery journey. Protein, for example, is vital for tissue repair and immune function. Patients may need higher protein intake to aid in healing and maintain muscle mass, especially if they experience weight loss or muscle wasting. Sources of high-quality protein include lean meats, poultry, fish, eggs, dairy products, legumes, and tofu.

Another essential nutrient is antioxidants, which help protect cells from damage caused by free radicals. Fruits and vegetables are excellent sources of antioxidants, vitamins, and minerals. Including a variety of colorful produce in the diet can provide a range of nutrients beneficial for overall health and immune support.

Foods rich in vitamins A, C, and E, as well as selenium and zinc, are particularly valuable for their antioxidant properties.

Omega-3 fatty acids are also important for oral cancer patients, as they have anti-inflammatory effects and may help reduce treatment-related side effects such as inflammation and mucositis.

 Fatty fish like salmon, mackerel, and sardines are rich in omega-3s, as are flaxseeds, chia seeds, and walnuts. Incorporating these foods into the diet can contribute to a healthier inflammatory response and improved overall well-being.

In contrast, certain foods should be limited or avoided to manage symptoms and support recovery. Spicy, acidic, or rough-textured foods can irritate the mouth and throat, leading to discomfort and potential complications. Foods that are too hot or too cold may also be challenging for patients with oral cancer, so it's important to find a balance of temperatures that are tolerable.

Additionally, foods high in sugar and refined carbohydrates should be limited, as they can contribute to inflammation, compromise immune function, and potentially fuel cancer growth. Opting for whole grains, fruits, and vegetables as sources of carbohydrates can provide fiber, vitamins, and minerals while supporting stable blood sugar levels.

Hydration is another critical aspect of nutrition for oral cancer patients. Adequate fluid intake helps prevent dehydration, supports saliva production, and facilitates swallowing. However, some patients may experience difficulty swallowing liquids, requiring modifications such as thickened beverages or using straws to assist with drinking.

In summary, nutrition plays a vital role in supporting oral cancer patients throughout their recovery process. A well-balanced diet rich in protein, antioxidants, omega-3 fatty acids, and hydration can help optimize treatment outcomes, manage symptoms, and improve overall quality of life. By understanding the importance of nutrition and making informed dietary choices, patients can enhance their resilience and well-being in the face of oral cancer challenges.

CHAPTER 2
Breakfasts For Oral Cancer Recovery

Energizing Smoothies and Juices

When it comes to breakfasts for oral cancer recovery, energizing smoothies and juices play a vital role in providing essential nutrients while being gentle on the digestive system.

These beverages are not only easy to consume but also packed with vitamins, minerals, and antioxidants that support the body's healing process.

Energizing smoothies often combine a variety of fruits and vegetables, along with protein sources such as yogurt or plant-based protein powders. They can be customized based on individual preferences and dietary needs. For oral cancer patients, it's crucial to include ingredients that are soft and easy to swallow, such as bananas, avocados, berries, and cooked vegetables. Adding liquids like almond milk, coconut water, or herbal teas helps in achieving the desired consistency and hydration.

The advantage of smoothies lies in their versatility. They can be enriched with superfoods like chia seeds, flaxseeds, or spirulina for added nutritional benefits. These ingredients not only boost energy levels but also aid in overall well-being. Additionally, incorporating healthy fats from sources like nuts or nut butters provides essential fatty acids that support brain health and immune function.

Similarly, juices are another excellent option for breakfast during oral cancer recovery. Freshly squeezed juices from fruits and vegetables offer a concentrated dose of vitamins and minerals. Carrot, beetroot, apple, and leafy greens like spinach or kale are common ingredients in healing juices. These ingredients are rich in antioxidants, which help combat inflammation and promote tissue repair.

It's essential to note that while juices can be nutrient-dense, they may lack fiber compared to whole fruits and vegetables. Therefore, a balanced approach that includes both smoothies and juices ensures a comprehensive nutrient intake. Moreover, using a high-quality blender or juicer ensures that the beverages are smooth and easy to swallow, maintaining comfort during meals.

energizing smoothies and juices are valuable additions to the breakfast routine of oral cancer patients. They provide essential nutrients, hydration, and energy while being gentle on the mouth and digestive system. By incorporating a variety of ingredients and superfoods, these beverages contribute to overall health and well-being during the recovery process.

Nutrient-Packed Breakfast Bowls

Nutrient-packed breakfast bowls offer a wholesome and satisfying start to the day, especially for individuals recovering from oral cancer.

These bowls are versatile, allowing for a combination of nutrient-rich ingredients that support healing and provide essential nutrients for overall well-being.

One popular option for breakfast bowls is a smoothie bowl, which combines the goodness of a smoothie with the texture of a thick porridge.

This bowl typically includes a base of blended fruits or vegetables, such as bananas, berries, or spinach, mixed with a liquid like almond milk or coconut water. Toppings such as granola, nuts, seeds, and fresh fruits add crunch, flavor, and additional nutrients.

Another variation of nutrient-packed breakfast bowls includes oatmeal or quinoa bowls. These grains are cooked with milk or water to a creamy consistency and then topped with fruits, nuts, seeds, and a drizzle of honey or maple syrup.

The advantage of using grains like oats or quinoa is their fiber content, which supports digestion and helps maintain stable blood sugar levels.

For oral cancer patients, it's essential to choose soft and easy-to-swallow ingredients for breakfast bowls. Cooked fruits like apples or pears, mashed bananas, and steamed vegetables can be incorporated into the bowls for added nutrition. Using creamy toppings like Greek yogurt or avocado adds a smooth texture and provides healthy fats and protein.

Moreover, nutrient-packed breakfast bowls can be customized to meet specific dietary requirements. For example, adding protein sources such as tofu, cottage cheese, or hemp seeds enhances satiety and supports muscle recovery. Including anti-inflammatory ingredients like turmeric, ginger, or green tea powder adds a therapeutic touch to the bowls, aiding in the healing process.

nutrient-packed breakfast bowls offer a delicious and nutritious option for oral cancer recovery. By combining a variety of soft and easy-to-digest ingredients, these bowls provide essential nutrients, fiber, and hydration to support overall health and well-being. Customizable and satisfying, they make breakfast a nourishing and enjoyable experience for patients on the road to recovery.

Healing porridges and oatmeal varieties are comforting and nutrient-rich breakfast options that support oral cancer recovery. These warm and soothing dishes are gentle on the digestive system while providing essential nutrients, fiber, and energy to kick-start the day.

Porridges can be made from a variety of grains, such as oats, quinoa, millet, or rice. Oats, in particular, are a popular choice due to their high fiber content and creamy texture when cooked.

To prepare healing porridges, the grains are cooked with milk or water until soft and then flavored with spices like cinnamon, nutmeg, or cardamom for added warmth and flavor.

For oral cancer patients, it's essential to choose ingredients that are easy to chew and swallow. Therefore, incorporating cooked fruits like apples, pears, or berries into the porridge adds natural sweetness and nutritional value. Additionally, adding protein sources such as nut butter, chia seeds, or Greek yogurt increases the protein content and aids in muscle repair and recovery.

Oatmeal varieties offer a versatile canvas for creating nourishing breakfast options. Overnight oats, for example, involve soaking oats in liquid (such as milk, yogurt, or plant-based alternatives) overnight, resulting in a soft and creamy texture by morning. Toppings such as fruits, nuts, seeds, and honey or maple syrup can be added before serving for a delicious and nutrient-packed meal.

The key to creating healing porridges and oatmeal varieties lies in the choice of ingredients and preparation methods. Using whole grains ensures a good source of complex carbohydrates, which provide sustained energy throughout the morning. Including fruits and protein-rich additions enhances the nutritional profile and supports the body's healing process.

Healing porridges and oatmeal varieties are wholesome and comforting breakfast choices for oral cancer recovery. By selecting soft and nutrient-rich ingredients, these dishes provide essential nutrients, fiber, and energy to fuel the day ahead. Customizable and delicious, they make breakfast a nourishing and enjoyable part of the recovery journey.

CHAPTER 3
Wholesome Main Dishes

Creating wholesome main dishes for recovery involves careful consideration of ingredients that provide essential nutrients and promote healing. Lean protein options are vital for supporting muscle repair and overall recovery. These proteins should be lean, meaning they have lower fat content while still providing ample protein to aid in tissue regeneration. Examples of lean proteins include chicken breast, turkey, fish like salmon or tilapia, and plant-based sources like tofu or tempeh.

Incorporating healing grains and legumes adds complexity and depth to main dishes while offering a range of nutrients such as fiber, vitamins, and minerals. Whole grains like quinoa, brown rice, and barley are excellent choices as they provide sustained energy and support digestive health. Legumes such as lentils, chickpeas, and black beans not only contribute protein but also fiber and antioxidants, enhancing the nutritional profile of the dish.

Vegetable-centric main courses are a cornerstone of a wholesome recovery meal. Vegetables provide a plethora of vitamins, minerals, and phytonutrients that support overall health and healing. Including a variety of colorful vegetables ensures a diverse array of nutrients, with options like leafy greens, cruciferous vegetables (broccoli, cauliflower), root vegetables (carrots, sweet potatoes), and nightshades (bell peppers, tomatoes) offering different benefits.

When preparing lean protein options, it's important to consider cooking methods that retain their nutritional value while enhancing flavor.

Grilling, baking, or steaming are healthier alternatives to frying, as they minimize added fats and preserve the natural goodness of the ingredients. Marinating proteins with herbs, spices, and healthy oils can also enhance their taste without compromising their nutritional integrity.

Healing grains and legumes can be incorporated into main dishes in various ways. For example, a quinoa salad with roasted vegetables and grilled chicken provides a balanced meal rich in protein, fiber, and antioxidants. Similarly, a lentil stew with whole grain bread offers a comforting and nutrient-dense option for recovery meals. Experimenting with different combinations and cooking techniques can keep main dishes interesting and satisfying.

Vegetable-centric main courses can be the highlight of a recovery meal, showcasing the vibrant colors and flavors of seasonal produce. Stir-fries with a colorful mix of vegetables and lean protein, vegetable-based curries served with whole grain rice, or stuffed bell peppers filled with quinoa and beans are just a few examples of nutrient-rich and delicious options. Including a variety of herbs, spices, and healthy fats like olive oil or avocado can elevate the taste while adding beneficial nutrients.

Overall, creating wholesome main dishes for recovery involves a thoughtful approach to ingredient selection, cooking methods, and flavor combinations. By focusing on lean protein options, healing grains and legumes, and vegetable-centric main courses, it's possible to design meals that nourish the body, support healing, and delight the palate.

CHAPTER 4
Brain-Boosting Salads And Dressings

Brain-boosting salads and dressings are not only delicious but also play a crucial role in promoting overall brain health. These salads are packed with nutrients that support cognitive function and may even have cancer-fighting properties.

By incorporating a variety of colorful fruits, vegetables, nuts, seeds, and healthy fats into your salads, you can create flavorful and nutritious meals that nourish both your body and mind.

One of the key components of brain-boosting salads is the inclusion of cancer-fighting ingredients. These ingredients often include dark leafy greens like kale, spinach, and arugula, which are rich in antioxidants such as vitamin C, vitamin E, and beta-carotene. These antioxidants help protect brain cells from oxidative stress and may reduce the risk of developing certain types of cancer.

Additionally, cruciferous vegetables like broccoli, cauliflower, and Brussels sprouts contain compounds that have been shown to inhibit the growth of cancer cells.

In addition to vegetables, brain-boosting salads often feature fruits that are high in antioxidants and other beneficial compounds. Berries, such as blueberries, strawberries, and raspberries, are particularly potent in this regard.

They contain flavonoids and polyphenols that have anti-inflammatory and neuroprotective effects, helping to maintain brain health and reduce the risk of cognitive decline.

Nuts and seeds are another important component of brain-boosting salads. They are rich in omega-3 fatty acids, which are essential for brain function and have been linked to a lower risk of Alzheimer's disease and other neurodegenerative disorders. Walnuts, almonds, flaxseeds, and chia seeds are excellent choices for adding a crunchy texture and a dose of healthy fats to your salads.

To enhance the flavor of brain-boosting salads, homemade dressings and vinaigrettes are often used. These dressings not only add taste but also provide additional nutrients and healthy fats.

Olive oil, for example, is a staple in Mediterranean-style dressings and is rich in monounsaturated fats, which are beneficial for heart and brain health. Including herbs and spices like basil, oregano, turmeric, and ginger in dressings can further boost their antioxidant and anti-inflammatory properties.

Creating brain-boosting salads and dressings at home allows for customization based on personal preferences and nutritional needs. You can experiment with different combinations of ingredients to create salads that are not only nutritious but also satisfying and enjoyable to eat. Incorporating a variety of textures, flavors, and colors not only makes the salads visually appealing but also ensures a diverse range of nutrients.

Brain-boosting salads and dressings are a delicious and nutritious way to support cognitive function and promote overall brain health.

By including cancer-fighting ingredients like dark leafy greens, berries, nuts, and seeds, as well as homemade dressings and vinaigrettes rich in healthy fats and antioxidants, you can create meals that nourish your body and mind. Experimenting with different ingredients and flavors allows for creativity in the kitchen while reaping the numerous health benefits of these brain-boosting foods.

CHAPTER 5
Nourishing Soups And Stews

Nourishing soups and stews hold a special place in culinary traditions across cultures, often embodying the essence of comfort and nourishment. These dishes not only satisfy the palate but also provide a wealth of health benefits when crafted with thoughtful ingredients and cooking techniques. Let's delve into the concepts surrounding nourishing soups and stews, exploring their role in promoting well-being and culinary enjoyment.

Soups and stews have long been celebrated for their ability to soothe the soul and support overall health, particularly during colder seasons or times of convalescence. The concept of nourishing soups goes beyond mere sustenance; it encompasses a culinary philosophy that prioritizes wholesome ingredients and slow cooking methods to extract maximum flavor and nutrition. From ancient healing broths to contemporary gourmet creations, soups have evolved into versatile culinary canvases that accommodate various dietary preferences and nutritional needs.

One of the key aspects of nourishing soups is their use of immune-boosting ingredients. These include but are not limited to:

1.   Broths and Stocks: The foundation of many nourishing soups and stews, homemade broths and stocks are rich in minerals, collagen, and amino acids that support gut health and immune function. Bone broths, in particular, are prized for their nutrient density and ability to strengthen the body's defenses.

2.   Vegetables: Colorful and diverse vegetables such as carrots, spinach, kale, bell peppers, and mushrooms not only lend flavor and texture to soups but also provide an array of vitamins, antioxidants, and phytonutrients that bolster immune resilience.

3.	Herbs and Spices: Incorporating herbs like thyme, rosemary, oregano, and spices such as turmeric, ginger, and garlic adds depth of flavor and potent anti-inflammatory, antimicrobial properties to soups, enhancing their immune-boosting potential.

4.	Protein Sources: Whether from animal or plant-based sources, adding protein-rich ingredients like chicken, beans, lentils, tofu, or quinoa to soups and stews not only increases satiety but also supports muscle repair and overall immune health.

5.	Healthy Fats: Including sources of healthy fats such as olive oil, avocado, or coconut milk not only enhances the creamy texture of soups but also aids in nutrient absorption and provides essential fatty acids vital for immune function.

In crafting comforting soups with immune-boosting ingredients, chefs and home cooks alike have the opportunity to experiment with flavors, textures, and nutrient profiles. From classic chicken noodle soup infused with herbs to hearty vegetable stews simmered in aromatic broths, the possibilities are as diverse as the ingredients themselves.

Turning our attention to hearty stews packed with nutrients, we enter a realm of culinary delights that marry robust flavors with wholesome goodness.

Stews are often characterized by slow cooking methods that allow ingredients to meld together, resulting in tender meats or vegetables bathed in rich, flavorful sauces.

The concept of nutrient-packed stews encompasses several key elements:

1.   Protein-Rich Ingredients: Stews traditionally feature protein-rich components such as beef, lamb, chicken, or seafood, providing essential amino acids and minerals crucial for muscle repair, hormone production, and overall vitality.

2.   Root Vegetables: The inclusion of root vegetables like potatoes, carrots, parsnips, and

turnips not only adds sweetness and depth to stews but also contributes complex carbohydrates, fiber, and a range of vitamins and minerals essential for energy metabolism and immune function.

3.   Legumes and Grains: To enhance the nutritional profile of stews, legumes such as lentils, chickpeas, or black beans can be incorporated, offering plant-based protein, fiber, and a host of micronutrients. Whole grains like barley, quinoa, or farro can also lend texture and nutritional density to stews.

4.   Aromatics and Flavor Enhancers: Utilizing aromatics such as onions, garlic, shallots, and leeks, along with flavor enhancers like tomato paste, Worcestershire sauce, soy sauce, or wine, elevates the taste profile of stews while providing antioxidant compounds and umami richness.

5.   Herbs and Spices: Herbs like thyme, bay leaves, sage, and spices such as paprika, cumin, coriander, and cinnamon play a vital role in

seasoning stews, contributing not just flavor complexity but also potential health benefits ranging from anti-inflammatory properties to digestive support.

6. Healthy Cooking Fats: Cooking stews in healthy fats like olive oil, ghee, or coconut oil not only enhances the mouthfeel and richness of the dish but also aids in the absorption of fat-soluble vitamins and promotes satiety.

The process of creating nutrient-packed stews involves layering flavors, balancing textures, and allowing ingredients to meld together harmoniously during the cooking process.

Whether simmered on the stovetop, slow-cooked in a Dutch oven, or prepared in a pressure cooker, stews offer a comforting and nutrient-dense dining experience that satisfies both the palate and the body's nutritional needs.

Nourishing soups and stews represent more than just meals; they embody a culinary tradition rooted in the art of nourishment, healing, and sensory pleasure.

By incorporating immune-boosting ingredients into comforting soups and nutrient-packed elements into hearty stews, individuals can elevate their culinary repertoire while supporting their well-being through wholesome, flavorful dishes.

CHAPTER 6
Memory-Enhancing Sandwiches And Wraps

Memory-Enhancing Sandwiches and Wraps are not just convenient meal options; they can also be power-packed with nutrients that support brain health and cognitive function. These culinary delights offer a delightful blend of flavors and textures, making them a popular choice for busy individuals looking for a quick yet nourishing meal. Let's delve into the concepts surrounding Memory-Enhancing Sandwiches and Wraps, exploring their ingredients, nutritional benefits, and creative fillings that contribute to a wholesome eating experience.

One of the key aspects of Memory-Enhancing Sandwiches and Wraps is their versatility. They can be customized to suit various dietary preferences and nutritional needs. Whether you prefer a classic sandwich with whole grain bread or a trendy wrap with a gluten-free alternative, there are endless possibilities to explore. Incorporating a variety of ingredients such as lean proteins, fresh vegetables, healthy fats, and brain-boosting herbs and spices is fundamental in creating a balanced and flavorful sandwich or wrap.

Starting with the bread or wrap itself, opting for whole grain varieties adds fiber, vitamins, and minerals to the meal. These complex carbohydrates provide a steady release of energy, keeping you satiated and focused for longer periods. Additionally, whole grains contain phytonutrients and antioxidants that support overall health, including brain function. Alternatives like whole wheat, spelt, or gluten-free options like quinoa or brown rice wraps offer diversity and cater to different dietary needs.

The fillings of Memory-Enhancing Sandwiches and Wraps play a crucial role in enhancing their nutritional value. Including lean proteins such as grilled chicken, turkey, tofu, or legumes like chickpeas or black beans provides essential amino acids necessary for neurotransmitter synthesis. These proteins also contribute to satiety and muscle maintenance, supporting overall well-being. Combining proteins with colorful vegetables like leafy greens, tomatoes, bell peppers, cucumbers, and avocados adds vitamins, minerals, and antioxidants to the meal.

Incorporating healthy fats is another aspect that sets Memory-Enhancing Sandwiches and Wraps apart. Avocado slices, olive oil-based dressings, or spreads like hummus or nut butter not only add creaminess and flavor but also provide omega-3 fatty acids and monounsaturated fats that are beneficial for brain health. Omega-3s, in particular, are known for their anti-inflammatory properties and role in cognitive function, making them a valuable addition to any brain-boosting meal.

Herbs, spices, and condiments are the finishing touches that elevate the taste and nutritional profile of Memory-Enhancing Sandwiches and Wraps. Fresh herbs like basil, cilantro, or mint not only add a burst of flavor but also contain antioxidants that protect against oxidative stress. Spices such as turmeric, cumin, and cinnamon offer anti-inflammatory and neuroprotective benefits, enhancing the overall wellness aspect of the meal. Opting for homemade dressings and spreads allows for better control of ingredients, reducing added sugars, sodium, and artificial additives.

Creativity knows no bounds when it comes to filling options for Memory-Enhancing Sandwiches and Wraps. From traditional combinations like turkey and cranberry sauce to exotic flavors like Thai peanut chicken wraps or Mediterranean veggie sandwiches, the choices are endless. Incorporating superfoods like kale, spinach, blueberries, or walnuts adds an extra nutritional punch. Experimenting with different textures, temperatures (think grilled veggies or warm fillings), and international cuisines keeps the meal experience exciting and enjoyable.

Meal planning and preparation play a significant role in incorporating Memory-Enhancing Sandwiches and Wraps into a balanced diet.

Batch cooking proteins, chopping vegetables in advance, and storing homemade dressings or spreads facilitate quick assembly during busy days. Preparing a variety of fillings allows for meal diversity throughout the week, ensuring a nutrient-rich diet without compromising on taste or convenience.

Pairing Memory-Enhancing Sandwiches and Wraps with complementary sides further enhances their nutritional value. Fresh fruit, raw veggies with dip, whole grain crackers, or a small portion of soup or salad create a well-rounded meal. Hydration is also essential for cognitive function, so including water, herbal teas, or infused water with fruits and herbs completes the dining experience.

Memory-Enhancing Sandwiches and Wraps offer a delightful fusion of flavors, textures, and nutrients that contribute to optimal brain health and cognitive function. By choosing wholesome ingredients, balancing macronutrients, and incorporating brain-boosting elements like lean proteins, healthy fats, colorful vegetables, and spices, these meals become more than just a quick bite—they become a nourishing and enjoyable part of a balanced diet. Embracing creativity in fillings and meal preparation adds excitement to everyday dining while supporting overall well-being.

CHAPTER 7
Snacks And Small Bites

Snacks and Small Bites are crucial elements in a balanced and health-conscious diet, offering quick energy boosts and satisfying hunger pangs between meals. When it comes to choosing snacks, the focus should be on both convenience and nutritional value, especially for individuals on a cancer recovery journey or seeking to prevent cancer through dietary choices.

This segment delves into the intricacies of crafting snacks and small bites that not only provide a burst of energy but also possess cancer-fighting properties, making them a valuable addition to daily nutrition.

Quick and healthy snacks play a vital role in maintaining energy levels throughout the day. These snacks are designed to be easily prepared, requiring minimal time and effort, which is particularly beneficial for busy individuals or those managing cancer-related fatigue.

Incorporating a variety of nutrient-dense ingredients into quick snacks ensures a balanced intake of essential nutrients, supporting overall health and well-being. Examples of such snacks include fresh fruit slices paired with nut butter or yogurt, whole-grain crackers with hummus, or a handful of nuts and seeds for a protein and fiber boost.

Bite-sized treats with cancer-fighting properties offer a unique opportunity to combine pleasure with purpose in snack choices. These snacks are not only delicious but also rich in antioxidants, vitamins, and minerals that contribute to a healthy immune system and may aid in cancer prevention or recovery. Incorporating ingredients like colorful fruits and vegetables, such as berries, citrus fruits, leafy greens, and cruciferous vegetables, into small bites creates a diverse array of flavors and textures while maximizing nutritional benefits.

Berries, known for their antioxidant properties due to high levels of polyphenols and vitamin C, can be incorporated into snacks like yogurt parfaits, smoothie bowls, or mixed into whole-grain muffin recipes. Citrus fruits, rich in vitamin C and flavonoids, can be used to make refreshing fruit salads or infused water for a hydrating and vitamin-packed snack option. Leafy greens like spinach, kale, and Swiss chard can be blended into smoothies or used as a base for nutrient-dense salads with added protein sources like grilled chicken or chickpeas.

Cruciferous vegetables such as broccoli, cauliflower, and Brussels sprouts are known for their cancer-fighting compounds, including sulforaphane and indole-3-carbinol.

These vegetables can be roasted with herbs and spices for a flavorful snack or incorporated into vegetable-based dips and spreads. Including a variety of colors and textures in snack preparations not only enhances visual appeal but also ensures a diverse intake of phytonutrients that support overall health and immune function.

In addition to fruits and vegetables, incorporating nuts, seeds, and whole grains into small bites adds essential nutrients like healthy fats, protein, fiber, and micronutrients.

Nuts like almonds, walnuts, and Brazil nuts are rich in omega-3 fatty acids, vitamin E, and minerals such as magnesium and selenium, offering heart-healthy benefits and antioxidant support.

Seeds like chia, flaxseed, and pumpkin seeds provide omega-3s, fiber, and plant-based protein, ideal for adding crunch and nutrition to snacks like energy balls, granola bars, or homemade trail mix.

Whole grains such as oats, quinoa, and brown rice offer complex carbohydrates, fiber, and B vitamins, promoting satiety and steady energy release. Including whole grains in snack recipes like homemade granola, whole-grain crackers, or whole-grain wraps filled with vegetables and lean protein sources enhances nutritional value and supports digestive health.

Choosing whole food ingredients and minimizing added sugars, refined flours, and artificial additives in snack preparations aligns with a cancer-fighting dietary approach focused on wholesome, nutrient-rich foods.

The synergy of ingredients in snacks and small bites is essential for optimizing health benefits, especially in the context of cancer prevention or recovery. Combining different food groups such as fruits, vegetables, lean proteins, healthy fats, and whole grains in snack options creates a balanced nutritional profile that supports immune function, promotes energy balance, and provides essential nutrients for cellular health and repair. Snacking mindfully, with an emphasis on nutrient density and variety, contributes to overall well-being and complements a cancer-aware lifestyle focused on holistic health practices.

CHAPTER 8
Beverages For Oral Cancer Recovery

Beverages play a crucial role in the recovery journey of patients dealing with oral cancer.

Not only do they contribute to hydration, but they can also provide essential nutrients and support overall well-being during treatment and recovery. Understanding the significance of beverages in oral cancer recovery involves delving into hydration tips tailored to the specific needs of these patients and exploring brain-enhancing drink recipes that can aid in cognitive function and overall health.

Hydration is a fundamental aspect of health for everyone, but it holds particular importance for individuals undergoing treatment for oral cancer. The side effects of cancer treatments such as chemotherapy and radiation therapy can often lead to dehydration, making it essential to focus on adequate fluid intake. Hydration tips for oral cancer patients revolve around strategies to maintain proper hydration levels despite potential challenges.

One key aspect of hydration for oral cancer patients is choosing the right fluids. Water is, of course, the primary recommendation due to its purity and lack of additives that may irritate sensitive oral tissues. However, for some patients experiencing taste changes or difficulty swallowing, plain water may not be appealing or easy to consume. In such cases, alternatives like infused water with fruits or herbs can add flavor without compromising hydration. It's essential to avoid beverages high in sugar, caffeine, or alcohol, as they can exacerbate dehydration or irritate oral tissues.

Another hydration tip is to consider the temperature of beverages. Cold liquids may be soothing for patients dealing with oral sores or inflammation, while warm or room-temperature fluids can be gentler on sensitive mouths.

Encouraging frequent sips throughout the day, rather than trying to consume large amounts at once, can also help maintain hydration without overwhelming the patient.

In addition to hydration, incorporating brain-enhancing drink recipes can further support oral cancer recovery by nourishing cognitive function and overall well-being. These recipes focus on ingredients known for their brain-boosting properties, such as antioxidants, omega-3 fatty acids, and vitamins that support neurological health.

One category of brain-enhancing drinks includes smoothies or shakes that combine fruits, vegetables, and other nutrient-rich ingredients.

For example, a blueberry and spinach smoothie can provide antioxidants and vitamins crucial for brain health, while adding a source of healthy fats like avocado or nuts can enhance nutrient absorption and satiety.

Herbal teas are another excellent option, offering hydration along with potential cognitive benefits. Teas like green tea, known for its antioxidant properties, or chamomile tea, which may have calming effects, can be soothing and beneficial for oral cancer patients. Adding ingredients like ginger or turmeric to teas not only enhances flavor but also provides anti-inflammatory and antioxidant benefits.

Incorporating beverages that include ingredients like coconut water or electrolyte-rich sports drinks can also help replenish essential minerals and maintain electrolyte balance, especially if treatment side effects include nausea, vomiting, or electrolyte imbalances.

Overall, the concept of beverages for oral cancer recovery encompasses not just hydration but also strategic choices that support overall health and well-being. By focusing on hydration tips tailored to the unique needs of oral cancer patients and exploring brain-enhancing drink recipes, caregivers and patients can work together to optimize nutritional support during treatment and recovery.

CHAPTER 9
Special Occasion Meals

Special occasion meals hold a unique place in our culinary traditions, marking moments of joy, connection, and celebration. These meals go beyond the everyday fare, often featuring elaborate dishes, rich flavors, and a sense of abundance that reflects the spirit of the occasion. Whether it's a holiday feast, a milestone celebration, or a gathering of loved ones, special occasion meals bring people together around the table to create lasting memories.

One of the defining characteristics of special occasion meals is their festive nature.

These meals are designed to be indulgent, with recipes that showcase the best of culinary creativity and craftsmanship. From elegant appetizers to decadent desserts, every aspect of the meal is carefully curated to delight the senses and create a sense of occasion. Festive recipes often feature premium ingredients, intricate cooking techniques, and stunning presentation, making them a feast for both the eyes and the palate.

When it comes to planning special occasion meals, consideration for dietary restrictions is essential. In today's diverse culinary landscape, people follow various dietary patterns and may have specific food allergies or intolerances. Therefore, adapting traditional festive recipes to accommodate these restrictions is both thoughtful and inclusive.

This can involve making substitutions, modifying cooking methods, or creating alternative dishes that still capture the essence of the celebration.

For example, a traditional holiday meal might include a roast turkey as the centerpiece.

To accommodate vegetarian guests, a delicious alternative could be a stuffed acorn squash with wild rice, cranberries, and pecans. This not only caters to dietary preferences but also adds a vibrant and flavorful option to the menu. Similarly, for those with gluten sensitivities, offering gluten-free versions of classic dishes like stuffing or dessert ensures that everyone can partake in the festivities without worry.

Another consideration is dietary choices such as veganism or paleo diets. For vegans, creative dishes like roasted vegetable Wellington or a plant-based charcuterie board can provide an impressive and satisfying meal.

Meanwhile, adhering to paleo principles might involve focusing on whole foods, lean proteins, and natural sweeteners, resulting in dishes like grilled salmon with roasted vegetables and a fruit-based dessert.

In addition to dietary restrictions, cultural and religious considerations also play a role in special occasion meals. For example, a Passover Seder meal would follow specific guidelines regarding ingredients and preparation methods to align with Jewish dietary laws. Similarly, Eid al-Fitr celebrations in the Muslim community often feature dishes like biryani, kebabs, and sweet treats like baklava, reflecting cultural traditions and culinary heritage.

Creating adaptations for dietary restrictions in special occasion meals requires creativity, attention to detail, and a deep understanding of flavor profiles and cooking techniques. It's about honoring traditions while embracing diversity and inclusivity at the table. By offering a variety of options that cater to different dietary needs, special occasion meals can truly be enjoyed by everyone, fostering a sense of unity and togetherness during these memorable moments.

CHAPTER 10
Meal Planning And Prep Strategies

Meal planning and preparation strategies play a crucial role in ensuring a healthy and balanced diet, especially for individuals with specific dietary needs. Whether it's catering to dietary restrictions, optimizing nutrient intake, or simplifying meal preparation, thoughtful planning and preparation can make a significant difference in maintaining a nutritious diet. In this discussion, we delve into the intricacies of meal planning and prep strategies, including weekly meal plans for different dietary needs, meal prep tips for convenience, and customizing meal plans for individual patients.

Weekly meal plans are structured plans that outline meals and snacks for each day of the week. These plans are designed to ensure a variety of nutrients while meeting specific dietary requirements. For example, a meal plan for someone following a vegan diet would focus on plant-based foods rich in proteins, vitamins, and minerals.

Similarly, a meal plan for someone with diabetes would prioritize low glycemic index foods to regulate blood sugar levels.

When creating weekly meal plans, it's essential to consider individual dietary needs. This includes allergies, intolerances, cultural preferences, and medical conditions. Customizing meal plans ensures that individuals receive adequate nutrition without compromising on taste or enjoyment.

For instance, someone with lactose intolerance would have dairy-free alternatives included in their meal plan, while someone with celiac disease would follow a gluten-free plan.

In addition to dietary needs, meal plans can also be tailored based on health goals. For example, a meal plan for weight management may focus on portion control and calorie balance, while a meal plan for muscle building may include higher protein and carbohydrate intake.

Customizing meal plans allows for personalized nutrition that supports overall health and wellness.

Meal prep tips are essential for busy individuals looking to maintain a healthy diet despite a hectic schedule. Effective meal prep involves preparing ingredients and meals in advance to streamline cooking and ensure access to nutritious food throughout the week.

One of the key strategies in meal prep is batch cooking, where large quantities of food are prepared at once and stored for later use. This not only saves time but also encourages healthy eating by having ready-to-eat meals available.

Another meal prep tip is to utilize versatile ingredients that can be used in multiple dishes.

For example, grilled chicken can be incorporated into salads, wraps, stir-fries, and pasta dishes, providing variety without requiring extensive cooking time. Prepping ingredients such as chopped vegetables, cooked grains, and marinated proteins makes assembling meals quick and convenient.

Furthermore, utilizing kitchen tools and appliances can streamline meal prep. Investing in a slow cooker, instant pot, or air fryer can simplify cooking processes and reduce hands-on time in the kitchen. Preparing meals in bulk and portioning them into individual servings also promotes portion control and prevents overeating.

Customizing meal plans for individual patients involves considering their unique nutritional needs, preferences, and health goals. This may require collaboration between healthcare professionals, such as registered dietitians, physicians, and chefs, to create tailored meal plans that align with medical recommendations and personal preferences. For example, a meal plan for someone recovering from surgery may focus on nutrient-dense foods that support healing and recovery, while a meal plan for an athlete may prioritize energy-dense meals for optimal performance.

Meal planning and preparation strategies are essential for promoting healthy eating habits and meeting individual dietary needs. Weekly meal plans tailored to different dietary requirements, meal prep tips for convenience, and customized meal plans for individual patients contribute to a well-rounded approach to nutrition.

By incorporating these strategies, individuals can enjoy nutritious and delicious meals while supporting their overall health and wellness.

Conclusion

This guide delves into the crucial intersection of nutrition and oral cancer recovery. We begin by understanding the nuances of oral cancer and its relationship with nutrition. Highlighting key nutrients and dietary considerations, we explore foods that aid in recovery while steering clear of those that may hinder progress.

Moving into specific meal categories, we offer a comprehensive range of options tailored for oral cancer patients.

Energizing breakfasts, wholesome main dishes rich in lean proteins and healing elements, brain-boosting salads, nourishing soups, memory-enhancing sandwiches, and snacks designed for quick energy are all included. We also delve into hydration strategies and brain-enhancing beverage recipes to support recovery.

Special occasion meals are not forgotten, with festive recipes that accommodate dietary restrictions. Lastly, we discuss effective meal planning and preparation strategics, offering customizable meal plans to meet varying needs. This holistic approach aims to empower patients with practical, nutritious choices throughout their oral cancer recovery journey.

www.ingramcontent.com/pod-product-compliance
Lightning Source LLC
Chambersburg PA
CBHW071217260726
48653CB00041B/889